AGE-DEFYING
STRENGTH EXERCISES

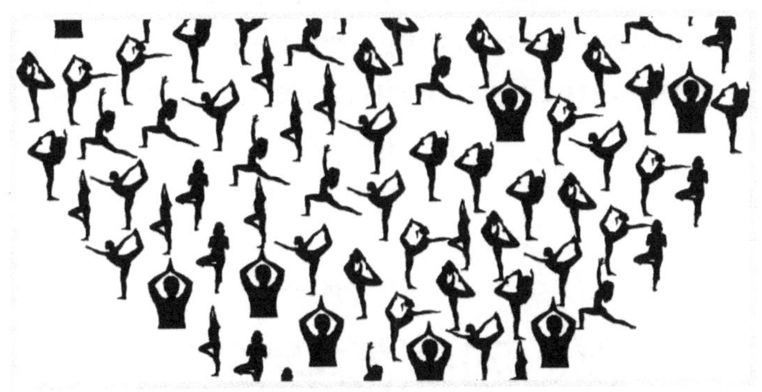

A Comprehensive Guide to Senior Strength Training and Active Aging

Curtis C. Figueroa

SCAN TO VIEW MORE BOOKS
SCAN ME!
CURTIS C. FIGUEROA
QR
Code

Table of Contents

CHAPTER FIVE - WORKOUT ROUTINES FOR

INTRODUCTION

In the serene town of Willowbrook, nestled amidst rolling hills and rustling leaves, lived Mr. Arthur Mitchell, a vibrant 70-year-old. Every morning, while the world was still draped in slumber, he embarked on a ritual, a dance with vitality that kept his spirit alight. Arthur, you see, was not just defying age; he was embracing it with a vigor that belied the passing years.

This book is a testament to Arthur and countless seniors like him who have discovered the secret to a fulfilling, joyful life exercise. In the pages that follow, we will explore the transformative power of physical activity, particularly for our cherished seniors.

The Importance of Exercising for Seniors

For seniors like Arthur, exercise is not merely a pastime; it's a lifeline. Regular exercise holds the power to bestow a multitude of benefits, from enhanced physical strength to improved mental clarity. It's a proven antidote to the wear and tear of aging, keeping muscles toned and joints supple. Beyond the physical, it fosters a sense of independence, allowing seniors to relish everyday activities with zest.

What is Exercise?

Exercise, in its essence, is intentional movement. It's a conscious effort to engage the body's muscles and systems in a way that enhances overall health. From brisk walks to heart-pumping workouts, exercise encompasses a broad spectrum of activities, each tailored to individual preferences and abilities.

What is Weight-Bearing Exercise?

Weight-bearing exercise is a cornerstone of any well-rounded fitness routine. It involves activities that force the body to work against gravity, such as walking, hiking, or lifting weights. This form of exercise promotes bone health, helps maintain muscle mass, and contributes to overall strength. It's particularly important for seniors, as it can reduce the risk of osteoporosis and fractures, ensuring a sturdy foundation for an active life.

The Importance of Exercise for Seniors

In the golden years, when life's pace may slow, the importance of exercise for seniors cannot be overstated. It's the elixir of longevity, the secret to maintaining independence, and the key to embracing every sunrise with enthusiasm. This book is a guide, a friend, and a source of inspiration, dedicated to seniors like Arthur Mitchell, who prove that age is but a number and that the path to vibrant health begins with a single step, a single exercise, and a world of possibilities.

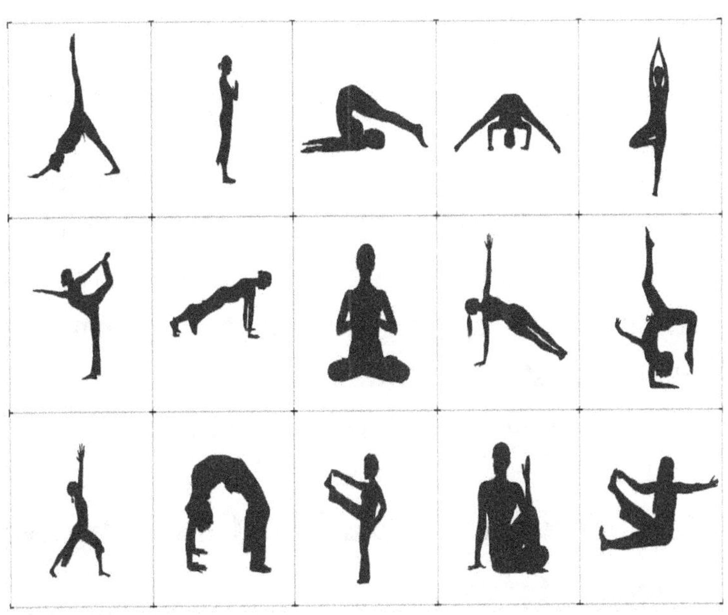

CHAPTER ONE - BENEFITS OF STRENGTH TRAINING FOR SENIORS

In the journey towards a healthier and more fulfilling senior life, embracing strength training is akin to discovering a treasure trove of wellness. This chapter illuminates the manifold benefits of strength training for seniors, delving into each aspect with expertise and insight.

How Strength Training Can Improve Glucose Metabolism

One of the most compelling reasons for seniors to engage in strength training is its remarkable effect on glucose metabolism. As we age, our bodies can become less sensitive to insulin, which leads to elevated blood sugar levels—a precursor to diabetes. Strength training, however, acts as a potent antidote. When we engage in resistance exercises, our muscles become more efficient at using glucose for energy. This enhanced efficiency not only stabilizes blood sugar levels but can also reduce the risk of developing type 2 diabetes.

Furthermore, strength training increases muscle mass. Muscles are voracious consumers of glucose, and the more muscle you have, the more effectively your body can regulate blood sugar. This means that seniors who make strength training a part of their routine can potentially improve their insulin sensitivity and reduce their reliance on medication to manage diabetes. It's a powerful tool in the arsenal against age-related metabolic changes. So, for seniors, embracing strength training isn't just about building muscle; it's about safeguarding metabolic health and paving the way for a more active and vibrant life.

Strength Training Can Help You Lose Weight

Weight management is a common concern as we age, and strength training emerges as a potent ally in this battle. Contrary to a popular misconception, strength training isn't just about bulking up; it's a strategic approach to shedding unwanted pounds.

Strength training promotes weight loss in several ways. First, it revs up your resting metabolic rate, meaning you burn more calories even when at rest. As you build lean muscle mass, your body requires more energy to maintain and repair these muscles, leading to a continuous calorie burn.

Secondly, it enhances fat loss. Muscles serve as metabolic furnaces, burning both glucose and fat for energy. Through consistent strength training, your body becomes proficient at utilizing fat stores for fuel, aiding in fat reduction.

Moreover, strength training positively influences body composition. Your body gets slimmer and more toned as you lose fat and increase muscle.

This not only contributes to a trimmer appearance but also to a healthier overall physique.

Crucially, strength training complements cardiovascular exercises, creating a well-rounded approach to weight management. The combination of increased muscle mass and cardiovascular conditioning can be particularly effective for seniors looking to shed excess weight, leading to better health and an improved quality of life.

Burning fats with Weight Training

For seniors seeking to shed unwanted body fat, weight training emerges as a powerful fat-burning tool. It's a misconception that fat loss primarily occurs through cardiovascular exercises; weight training plays a pivotal role in this endeavor.

Weight training, or resistance exercises, challenges your muscles, causing tiny tears that need repair. This repair process consumes calories, even after your workout is over. As a result, your body continues to burn fat for energy long after you've left the gym.

Moreover, weight training improves your muscle-to-fat ratio. As you build lean muscle mass, your body becomes more efficient at burning fat, as muscles are metabolically active and require energy for maintenance.

The benefits extend beyond just fat loss. Weight training helps preserve bone density, which is especially crucial for seniors, as it reduces the risk of osteoporosis. It also enhances balance and stability, decreasing the likelihood of falls and injuries.

Seniors should view weight training not as a means to bulk up but as a way to sculpt their bodies, reduce fat stores, and enhance overall health. When paired with a balanced diet and cardiovascular exercise, weight training is an indispensable component of a comprehensive approach to fat loss and improved well-being.

Can Strength Training Build Muscle?

The desire to maintain or build muscle might seem incompatible with the aging process, but the truth is that seniors can experience significant muscle gains through strength training. It's a myth that muscle-building is exclusive to the young; in fact, it's vital for seniors.

Strength training stimulates the creation of new muscle fibers, a process known as hypertrophy. This results in increased muscle mass, improved strength, and enhanced physical function. For seniors, these gains are not merely cosmetic but profoundly functional.

Building muscle as you age has numerous benefits. It improves mobility, making daily tasks easier and reducing the risk of injuries. Seniors who engage in strength training often find that they can maintain their independence for longer periods.

Furthermore, increased muscle mass boosts metabolism, which aids in weight management and glucose regulation. It also helps maintain bone density, a critical factor in preventing osteoporosis.

The key to successful muscle-building in seniors lies in proper guidance and consistency. Strength training, when performed with the right technique and progressively challenging loads, can lead to remarkable gains, improving overall health and vitality. It's a testament to the body's remarkable capacity for adaptation and regeneration, regardless of age.

Strength Training Guidelines

Before delving into the specifics of strength training, it's essential to establish some fundamental guidelines, especially for seniors. Strength training offers numerous benefits, but safety and precision are paramount.

Consult Your Healthcare Provider: Prior to embarking on a strength training regimen, consult your healthcare provider, especially if you have underlying health concerns. They can provide guidance and ensure your exercise plan aligns with your medical history and current condition.

Start Light and Progress Gradually: Seniors should begin with light resistance and gradually increase intensity over time. This progressive approach minimizes the risk of injury while allowing for steady strength gains.

Proper Technique Matters: Correct form is crucial to prevent injuries and maximize results. Consider working with a certified trainer, at least initially, to learn proper technique for each exercise.

Balance is Key: Include exercises that target various muscle groups to promote balance and functional strength. Don't focus solely on one area of the body.

Pay Attention to Your Body: Be aware of the indications that your body is giving you. When you experience pain or discomfort that is more intense than ordinary muscle soreness, stop completing the exercise.

Rest and recovery: Allow adequate time between workouts for your muscles to recover. It takes time for muscles to build and recuperate.

Nutrition Matters: A balanced diet that includes adequate protein is essential to support muscle growth and recovery.

Stay Hydrated: Proper hydration is often overlooked but crucial for overall health and muscle function.

Incorporating these guidelines into your strength training routine ensures that you reap the full benefits of this exercise modality while minimizing the risk of injury. Strength training, when approached wisely, can be a lifelong source of physical vitality for seniors.

Strength Training For Weight Loss

For seniors on a weight loss journey, strength training serves as a valuable companion to a healthier lifestyle. While cardio exercises burn calories during the activity, strength training contributes to weight loss in a unique and essential way.

Strength training boosts metabolism, causing the body to burn more calories at rest. The more lean muscle mass you possess, the higher your resting metabolic rate becomes. This means that even when you're not exercising, your body is efficiently burning calories, making it easier to create a calorie deficit, a fundamental requirement for weight loss.

Furthermore, strength training helps preserve existing muscle mass during periods of calorie restriction. While dieting, the body tends to burn both fat and muscle for energy. However, strength training signals the body to prioritize fat over muscle, helping you retain the lean mass that's crucial for a healthy metabolism.

Seniors embarking on a weight loss journey should incorporate both strength training and cardio exercises into their routine. Together, these approaches create a powerful synergy for shedding pounds and maintaining a healthy weight. It's an effective strategy that not only supports weight loss but also enhances overall fitness and well-being as you age.

Strength Training for Runners

For seniors with a passion for running or those considering taking up this cardiovascular activity, incorporating strength training into your regimen can be a game-changer. It's a dynamic duo that can help you run with ease and minimize the risk of injury.

Strength training provides several advantages for runners, especially seniors. First and foremost, it enhances muscular endurance. This means your leg muscles can maintain the necessary power output during longer runs, reducing fatigue.

Additionally, strength training improves joint stability and flexibility. Seniors often grapple with joint issues, but targeted strength training exercises can strengthen the supporting structures around your joints, reducing the likelihood of injuries like sprains or strains.

Furthermore, strength training increases overall body strength, which translates into more efficient running mechanics. It helps you maintain proper posture and form throughout your runs, which is critical for injury prevention and overall running performance.

For senior runners, a well-rounded fitness routine that combines running with strength training can extend your running career, allowing you to continue enjoying the physical and mental benefits of this beloved activity. It's an investment in your health, longevity, and the sheer joy of running.

Strength Training Importance

In the realm of senior fitness, the importance of strength training cannot be overstated. As we age, the natural process of muscle loss, known as sarcopenia, can have far-reaching implications for our health and quality of life. Strength training stands as a potent antidote to this decline.

One of the most significant benefits of strength training for seniors is its ability to counteract muscle loss. Regular resistance exercises stimulate the growth of new muscle fibers, promoting increased muscle mass and strength. This, in turn, enhances mobility, making everyday tasks easier to accomplish and reducing the risk of falls and fractures.

Beyond muscle preservation, strength training also contributes to better metabolic health. It boosts metabolism, helping to control body weight and improve glucose metabolism. For seniors, this can be a crucial factor in maintaining overall health and preventing conditions like type 2 diabetes.

Strength training is also renowned for its bone-building benefits. By subjecting bones to controlled stress through resistance exercises, it stimulates bone density improvements, reducing the risk of osteoporosis and fractures.

In essence, strength training is the cornerstone of senior fitness, offering a multitude of advantages that span from improved muscle mass and bone density to enhanced metabolic health. It's a key player in the pursuit of a vibrant and active senior life.

Strength Training is Good for the Heart

As seniors aspire to lead heart-healthy lives, it's imperative to recognize the pivotal role that strength training plays in cardiovascular well-being. While it's often associated with building muscle, it also offers substantial benefits for the heart and overall cardiovascular health.

One of the key advantages of strength training is its positive effect on blood pressure. Engaging in resistance exercises on a regular basis can lead to significant reductions in both systolic and diastolic blood pressure. Lower blood pressure translates to a reduced risk of heart disease, strokes, and related complications.

Strength training can also improve a person's cholesterol profile. It has been demonstrated to lower levels of low-density lipoprotein (LDL), or "bad" cholesterol, while increasing levels of high-density lipoprotein (HDL), or "good" cholesterol. This shift in cholesterol levels is conducive to a healthier cardiovascular system.

Strength training also promotes overall heart health by improving vascular function. It enhances the flexibility of blood vessels, which aids in better blood flow and reduces the risk of arterial stiffening, a common occurrence with age.

For seniors concerned about their heart health, incorporating strength training into their fitness routine is a wise choice.

It complements cardiovascular exercise, contributing to a comprehensive approach for maintaining a robust and resilient heart.

Strength Training is Best for Weight Loss

When it comes to weight management, especially for seniors, strength training emerges as the frontrunner in effectiveness and sustainability. While cardio exercises have their merits, strength training reigns supreme for long-term weight loss.

One of the primary reasons strength training is ideal for weight loss is its ability to increase resting metabolic rate. As you build lean muscle mass, your body becomes a more efficient calorie-burning machine, even when you're at rest. This metabolic boost continues well after your workout, helping to create a calorie deficit necessary for weight loss.

Moreover, strength training helps to preserve and even increase lean muscle mass during weight loss. When dieting, it's common for the body to break down both fat and muscle for energy. However, with strength training, your body prioritizes burning fat over muscle, preserving your muscle mass. This is crucial for maintaining a healthy metabolism and preventing the "yo-yo" effect of regaining lost weight.

Additionally, strength training enhances overall body composition. As you lose fat and build muscle, you'll achieve a leaner, more toned appearance. This not only contributes to a healthier weight but also boosts self-esteem and body confidence.

For seniors seeking sustainable weight loss, incorporating strength training into their fitness routine is a strategic and effective choice. It's a path to long-term success that positively impacts not only weight but overall health and vitality.

Strength Training Around Period

For seniors, incorporating strength training into their fitness routine, even during times of physical transition such as menopause for women, is a wise decision. Strength training offers unique benefits that can help alleviate some of the challenges associated with this phase of life.

Menopause often brings hormonal changes that can lead to weight gain and muscle loss. Strength training can counteract these effects by increasing muscle mass, which, as discussed earlier, raises resting metabolic rate and aids in weight management.

Furthermore, strength training helps with bone health, which is particularly important for women experiencing menopause. The decline in estrogen levels during menopause can lead to decreased bone density and an increased risk of osteoporosis. Strength training stimulates bone growth and density, reducing the likelihood of fractures and bone-related issues.

It's important to adapt strength training routines to individual needs and comfort levels during menopause. Working with a qualified trainer or fitness professional can help tailor exercises to address specific goals and potential challenges associated with this life stage.

In summary, strength training during menopause is not only safe but highly beneficial. It can mitigate weight gain, preserve muscle mass, improve bone density, and contribute to overall well-being during this natural transition.

CHAPTER TWO: GETTING STARTED WITH GENTLE STRENGTH TRAINING FOR SENIORS

As we age, maintaining physical strength and balance becomes increasingly essential for our overall well-being and independence. Gentle strength training exercises are an excellent way for seniors to enhance their muscular strength, improve balance, and reduce the risk of falls and injuries. This chapter introduces a series of exercises designed specifically for seniors, each with its unique set of benefits.

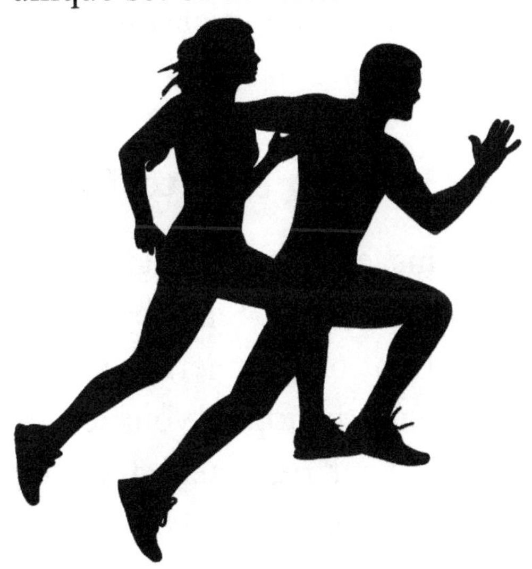

Exercise 1: Single Limb Stance

Procedure: Begin by standing behind a sturdy chair (one without wheels) and holding onto the back for support. Balance on your left foot while raising your right foot off the ground. Try to maintain this stance for as long as you can, then switch to balancing on your right foot. The goal is to eventually balance without holding onto the chair, aiming for up to a minute on each foot.

Health Advantage: This exercise primarily targets balance, which is crucial for preventing falls. It strengthens the muscles in your legs and core while improving stability.

Exercise 2: Walking Heel to Toe

Procedure: This exercise strengthens your legs and enhances balance. Start by placing your right foot in front of your left foot so that your right heel touches the top of your left toes. Shift your weight to your right heel, then to your left toes, and continue this heel-to-toe walking pattern for 20 steps.

Health Advantage: Walking heel to toe improves leg strength and coordination, making it easier to walk steadily without stumbling.

Exercise 3: Rock the Boat

Procedure: Stand with your feet hip-width apart, ensuring both are firmly planted on the ground. As you shift your weight to your right foot, steadily raise your left leg. Hold this position for as long as you can, up to 30 seconds, then return your left foot to the ground and switch to your right leg.
Health Advantage: Rock the Boat enhances balance and strengthens leg muscles, crucial for stability and fall prevention.

Exercise 4: Clock Reach

Procedure: Use a chair for support. Imagine yourself in the center of a clock, with 12 directly in front of you and 6 behind. Hold the chair with your left hand and extend your right arm toward 12. Move your arm to 3, then behind you to 6, returning to 3, and finally to 12. Keep your gaze straight ahead.

Health Advantage: Clock Reach enhances balance and coordination while targeting the muscles in your arms and shoulders.

Exercise 5: Back Leg Raises

Procedure: This exercise targets your lower back and buttocks. To begin, lean on a chair for support.. Lift your right leg slowly back, straightening it out without bending the knee or pointing the toes. Hold this position for one second, then gently lower your leg. Repeat this movement ten to fifteen times for each leg.
Health Advantage: Back leg raises strengthen the lower back and buttocks, improving posture and overall lower body strength.

Exercise 6: Single Limb Stance with Arm

Procedure: Stand with your feet together and your arms at your sides next to a chair. Lift your left hand over your head while slowly raising your left foot off the floor. Hold this position for ten seconds. Then, switch to your right side and repeat.

Health Advantage: This exercise enhances physical coordination and balance, working both upper and lower body muscles.

Exercise 7: Side Leg Raise

Procedure: This exercise targets the muscles on the sides of your hips and thighs. Stand behind a chair with your feet slightly apart. Slowly lift your right leg to the side while keeping your toe facing forward. Lower your right leg slowly. Repeat this exercise ten to fifteen times for each leg.
Health Advantage: Side leg raises help improve balance and strengthen the muscles responsible for stability during daily activities.

Exercise 8: Balancing Wand

Procedure: For this balance exercise, you'll need a cane or a stick (e.g., a broomstick with the broom head removed). Hold the stick so that the bottom is flat against the palm of your hand. The goal is to keep the stick upright for as long as possible while changing hands to work on balance skills for both sides of your body.

Health Advantage: The balancing wand exercise enhances overall balance and stability, reducing the risk of falls.

Exercise 9: Wall Pushups

Procedure: Stand at arm's length in front of a wall without any decorations or obstructions. Lean forward slightly and place your palms flat on the wall at shoulder height and shoulder-width apart. Keep your feet planted as you slowly bring your body towards the wall, then push yourself back so that your arms are straight. Repeat this movement twenty times.

Health Advantage: Wall pushups help strengthen the chest, shoulders, and triceps, improving upper body strength.

Exercise 10: Marching in Place

Procedure: Marching is an excellent balance exercise. Stand straight and lift your right knee as high as you can, then lower it. Alternately move your left leg in the same manner. Alternate between legs, lifting and lowering them twenty times.

Health Advantage
Marching in place improves balance, leg strength, and coordination.

These exercises are tailored to improve strength, balance, and overall physical well-being for seniors. Remember to consult your healthcare provider before starting any new exercise program, especially if you have underlying health conditions or concerns. Incorporating these exercises into your routine can help you maintain your independence and enjoy an active lifestyle as you age.

CHAPTER THREE - DIFFERENT APPROACHES TO STRENGTH TRAINING

Variety is the spice of life, and the same holds true for strength training. In this chapter, we explore diverse approaches to strength training, each offering unique benefits. Whether you prefer using equipment like resistance bands, dumbbells, or even opting for a minimalist no-equipment routine, there's a method that suits your preferences and goals.

Strength Training with Resistance Bands

Explanation: Resistance bands are versatile tools that provide consistent resistance throughout the movement. They come in different levels of resistance, making them suitable for beginners and advanced individuals alike. To use resistance bands effectively, anchor them securely and perform exercises that mimic traditional weightlifting movements, such as bicep curls, leg lifts, and chest presses. The bands add tension to your muscles, enhancing strength and endurance.

Tips: Choose the appropriate resistance level based on your fitness level. Progressively raise the resistance as your strength grows. To optimize performance and reduce the chance of injury, concentrate on maintaining good form throughout each exercise.

Strength Training with Dumbbells

Explanation: Dumbbells are classic tools for strength training, offering a wide range of exercises that target various muscle groups. They enable unilateral training, which aids in resolving muscular imbalances. Whether you're an advanced lifter or a beginner, dumbbell routines can be readily adapted to fit your fitness level.

Tips: Start with a weight that allows you to perform exercises with proper form. As your strength grows, progressively increase the weight. For best results, concentrate on a wide range of motion and controlled movements.

Strength Training with Bands:

Explanation: Similar to resistance bands, exercise bands provide varying degrees of resistance. They can be utilized for exercises for the upper and lower bodies. For those who have joint problems or injuries, exercise bands offer a comfortable solution.

Tips: Use bands that provide the appropriate resistance level for your fitness level. Securely anchor the bands to a stable surface. Maintain tension in the band throughout each movement and focus on controlled repetitions.

Strength Training with Weights:

Explanation: Free weights, such as barbells and dumbbells, offer functional strength training by engaging stabilizing muscles. Squats, deadlifts, and bench presses are examples of compound exercises that simultaneously engage several muscular groups.

Tips: Learn proper form for each exercise to prevent injuries. As your strength grows, progressively increase the weight.

. Incorporate a variety of free weight exercises to ensure balanced muscle development.

Strength Training with Kettlebell:

Explanation: Kettlebells combine cardiovascular and strength training benefits in one workout. Their unique design allows for dynamic movements like swings and snatches, engaging both upper and lower body muscles.

Tips: Master proper kettlebell form before attempting complex exercises.

Focus on hip hinge movements and maintain a strong core throughout the exercises.

Strength Training with No Equipment:

Explanation: No equipment? No problem. Bodyweight exercises like push-ups, squats, and planks are effective for strength training. Use your own weight as resistance throughout these workouts.

Tips: Perform bodyweight exercises with proper form and control. Modify exercises as needed to match your fitness level.

The journey to health and fitness is as diverse as the individuals embarking on it. Choosing the right strength training approach can make your fitness routine enjoyable and effective. Tailor your regimen to your goals and preferences, and remember that consistency and proper form are key to achieving the best results.

Strength Training Without Weights:

Explanation: Strength training without weights focuses on utilizing your body's resistance to build muscle and strength. Bodyweight exercises like squats, lunges, and push-ups are staples of this approach. These exercises can be performed virtually anywhere, making them convenient for at-home workouts or when you're on the go.

Tips: Pay attention to your form and technique during bodyweight exercises. Focus on controlled movements, and for added challenge, you can adjust the difficulty level by increasing repetitions or incorporating variations of the exercises.

Strength Training Without Bulking:

Explanation: Some individuals, particularly seniors, may be concerned about bulking up through strength training. It's essential to understand that strength training does not inherently lead to bulky muscles. In fact, it's an effective way to tone and sculpt the body without excessive muscle growth.

Tips: To avoid excessive muscle growth, use lighter weights or resistance bands with higher repetitions. Focus on full-body workouts that target multiple muscle groups and incorporate cardiovascular exercise to balance your fitness routine.

Strength Training Without Cardio:

Explanation: While cardio exercise is beneficial for overall health, it's not always a preferred choice. Strength training can provide a way to improve fitness without traditional cardio activities like running or cycling. Compound exercises such as squats, deadlifts, and kettlebell swings elevate the heart rate while building muscle.

Tips: Integrate compound movements into your strength training routine. Perform exercises in a circuit format with minimal rest between sets to increase cardiovascular engagement.

Strength Training Without Protein:

Explanation: While protein is crucial for muscle recovery and growth, you can engage in strength training without relying solely on protein supplementation. A balanced diet that includes lean protein sources like chicken, fish, tofu, and beans can provide the necessary nutrients for muscle repair.

Tips: Ensure you're meeting your daily protein needs through whole foods. Monitor your diet to include a variety of nutrient-rich foods to support your strength training efforts.

Strength Training Without Bulking Up:

Explanation: Building lean muscle through strength training is a common goal, but many individuals worry about bulking up excessively. The truth is that bulking up significantly requires specific training programs and nutrition plans designed for bodybuilders.

Tips: To avoid bulking up, focus on moderate resistance and higher repetitions. Incorporate bodyweight exercises and resistance bands into your routine for a more toned and defined physique.

Strength Training Without Shoes:

Explanation: While it's common to wear athletic shoes during strength training, some individuals prefer to go barefoot. Strength training without shoes allows for better connection with the ground and can improve balance and stability.

Tips: If you choose to train without shoes, ensure you're working out in a safe, clean environment. Consider using a gym mat for added comfort and hygiene.

Each of these approaches to strength training offers a unique perspective on fitness, catering to individual preferences and goals. The key to a successful strength training program is finding the method that aligns with your objectives, staying consistent, and prioritizing proper form and technique to maximize results while minimizing the risk of injury. Always get advice from a fitness expert or a medical specialist to choose the strategy that will work best for you.

CHAPTER FOUR - DEVELOPING THE HABIT OF WORKING OUT

The key to a successful fitness journey is consistency. In this chapter, we delve into the art of developing the habit of working out, specifically tailored to seniors. Establishing a routine, beginning with a solid start, and understanding essential warm-up and stretching practices are key elements for a sustainable workout habit.

How to Develop the Habit of Working Out:

Explanation: Establishing a habit requires intention and dedication. Start by establishing specific, attainable exercise objectives. Create a workout schedule that fits your lifestyle, whether it's in the morning, during lunch breaks, or in the evening. Consistency is more important than intensity. Begin with manageable workouts and gradually increase the duration and intensity as your habit solidifies.

Tips: Use a fitness journal to track your progress and celebrate your achievements, no matter how small they seem. Join a fitness group or find a training partner for accountability and encouragement. Keep your workouts enjoyable by trying various activities to discover what you love.

How Seniors Can Get Started:

Explanation: Starting a workout routine as a senior requires a thoughtful approach. Begin by consulting with your healthcare provider to ensure that exercise is safe for your specific health conditions. Once you receive the green light, consider working with a certified fitness trainer who specializes in senior fitness. They can design a tailored workout plan that aligns with your goals and limitations.

Certainly, developing a consistent exercise routine can be challenging, but with the right strategies, it becomes an attainable habit. Here are 10 tips to help you start an exercise routine and make it a lasting part of your life:

Start with Small Goals: Begin with achievable goals, even if it's just 10 minutes of exercise. Gradually increase the duration and intensity as you build confidence and stamina. Keep in mind that any activity is preferable to none.

Use a Smartwatch or Pedometer: Track your daily steps with a smartwatch or pedometer and aim for a target like 10,000 steps a day. Monitoring your progress can be motivating and help you stay on track.

Incorporate Exercise into Your Routine: Look for opportunities to exercise in your daily life. Perform exercises while watching TV, during commercial breaks, or while waiting for dinner to cook. It's about making the most of your time.

Whenever possible, take the stairs instead of the elevator or the escalator. It's a simple way to add physical activity to your day and improve cardiovascular health.

Increase Visibility: Place your workout gear or gym bag in a visible location, like the kitchen or living room. When you see it, it serves as a reminder and makes the decision to exercise more conscious.

Stay Consistent: Building a habit takes time, typically around a month. Be kind to yourself and persevere. Consistency is key to making exercise a natural part of your routine.

Set Goals: Sign up for a fitness challenge or race to give yourself a concrete goal to work towards. Having a target can boost motivation and keep you committed to your exercise routine.

Explore Different Types of Exercise: Find an activity you genuinely enjoy. There's a wide range of options, from running and weightlifting to swimming and team sports. Try several things until you find what you enjoy.

Schedule Your Workouts: Treat exercise as an important appointment by scheduling it in your calendar. Make it non-negotiable, just like any other commitment.

Experiment with Timing: Try different workout times to determine when you have the most energy and motivation. Don't rule out early morning routines; you might find they kickstart your day with a burst of energy.

Remember, the key to success is finding an exercise routine that fits your lifestyle and preferences. Start small, stay consistent, and gradually increase the challenge. Over time, exercise will become a natural and rewarding part of your daily life.

Tips: Start slow and gradually progress. Focus on functional fitness exercises that improve daily life activities. Don't be discouraged by initial challenges; consistency is the key to improvement.

How to Approach the Workout:

Explanation: A well-rounded workout includes strength training, cardiovascular exercise, flexibility work, and balance training. Balance these components to create a holistic fitness routine. Aim for at least 150 minutes per week of moderate-intensity aerobic exercise and at least two sessions per week of strength training.

Tips: Prioritize exercises that align with your goals and abilities. Listen to your body and make necessary modifications. Include exercises that improve mobility, joint health, and posture.

Dynamic Stretches and Static Stretches:
Explanation: Dynamic stretches involve active movements that increase blood flow and prepare your muscles for exercise. Examples include leg swings and arm circles. Static stretches are held for a period without movement and are typically performed at the end of a workout to improve flexibility.

Tips: Incorporate dynamic stretches into your warm-up routine to reduce the risk of injury. Save static stretches for post-workout to improve flexibility and prevent muscle soreness.

Warming-Up Exercises:

Explanation: Warming up is essential to increase blood flow, heart rate, and body temperature before engaging in more intense exercises. Start with light aerobic activities like brisk walking or cycling. Include dynamic stretches to loosen up joints and muscles.

Tips: Spend 5-10 minutes warming up before your workout. Gradually increase the intensity to match your workout's level of intensity. Focus on proper form during warming-up exercises.
Developing the habit of working out as a senior is an empowering journey that contributes to improved health and vitality. The key is to begin with realistic goals, consult professionals as needed, and prioritize a well-rounded fitness routine that includes warm-up and stretching

practices. Stay patient and persistent, and remember that every workout brings you closer to your fitness goals.

Warming Up Stretching for Seniors and the Elderly

Warming up and stretching are essential components of any exercise routine, especially for seniors and the elderly. These exercises help improve flexibility, range of motion, and joint mobility while reducing the risk of injury. Let's delve into some warming up stretching exercises tailored for older adults:

1. Ankle Circles

Purpose: This exercise is designed to improve the range of motion of the ankle and foot, making it particularly useful for seniors experiencing ankle stiffness or swelling.

Step 1: Sit comfortably in your chair, ensuring stability and relaxation.

Step 2: Extend your right leg gently or lightly cross it over the left. Now, circle your right ankle ten times in each direction. The left leg should be used for the same motions.

Breathing
Maintain normal breathing, inhaling through the nose and exhaling through the mouth.

Tips: If you've had recent hip surgery, consult your doctor or physical therapist for any movement precautions. Simply extend your knee for the action if you suffer numbness in your foot while performing this exercise. For an added challenge, you can try extending both legs out simultaneously.

These ankle circles serve as an excellent warm-up for the ankle joint, calf muscles, shin muscles, and feet.

2. Additional Stretching Exercises for Seniors
In addition to ankle circles, seniors can benefit from a range of stretching exercises:

Seated Lifts: Improve hip and leg range of motion while stabilizing the lower back and pelvis.

Standing Quadriceps Stretch: Enhance hip and knee flexibility, leading to improved standing posture.

Back Stretch: Increase spine and trunk range of motion, making bending and reaching easier.

Inner Thigh Stretch: Improve hip and thigh mobility for better standing, walking, and stepping ability.

Calf Stretch: Target calf muscles and heel cord flexibility, enhancing knee straightening capability.

Hip Side Stretch: Ideal for stretching the side hip area, improving hip range of motion, and enhancing balance.

Hip Rotation Stretch: Increase hip range of motion for everyday activities like getting in and out of a car or stepping into a bath.

Soleus Stretch: Work on the flexibility of the deep calf muscle, benefiting overall lower body flexibility.

Hamstring Stretch: Increase forward-reaching capability and flexibility in the low back and legs.

Knee To Chest: Stretch knee and hip joints while promoting low back flexibility.

Ankle Stretch: Maintain ankle flexibility for better walking and standing, particularly beneficial for those with knee and hip stiffness.

Warming up and stretching exercises are vital for seniors and the elderly to maintain and improve mobility, reduce the risk of falls, and enjoy a more active and independent lifestyle. Remember to consult with a healthcare provider or physical therapist before starting any new exercise routine, especially if you have specific health concerns or limitations.

CHAPTER FIVE - WORKOUT ROUTINES FOR SENIORS

In this chapter, we'll explore a variety of workout routines specifically designed for seniors to enhance strength, flexibility, balance, and overall well-being. These routines cater to different fitness levels, ensuring that everyone can find a routine that suits their abilities and goals.

10-Minute Workout Routines:

Explanation: These quick, effective workouts are perfect for those with busy schedules or limited time. They focus on maximizing results in just 10 minutes, providing a convenient way to stay active.

Tips: Choose a 10-minute routine that aligns with your fitness goals, whether it's strength, balance, or flexibility. Perform these routines as a daily habit to build consistency.

Sitting Workout:

Explanation: Ideal for seniors with mobility challenges, this seated workout allows you to exercise while comfortably seated in a chair. It focuses on gentle movements to improve strength and flexibility.

Tips: Ensure your chair is stable and positioned on a non-slip surface. Pay attention to proper posture and form throughout the seated workout.

Balance Workout:

Explanation: Balance is crucial for preventing falls and maintaining independence. This workout includes exercises specifically designed to enhance balance and stability.

Tips: Use a sturdy chair or wall for support during balance exercises, especially if you're new to this type of workout. Gradually increase the duration and intensity of balance exercises over time.

Beginner Standing Workout:

Explanation: This workout is tailored for beginners who want to transition from seated exercises to standing exercises.It emphasizes enhancing general strength and mobility.

Tips: Start with low-impact exercises and gradually increase the intensity as you gain confidence. Use proper footwear and ensure a safe workout environment.

Core-Focused Workout:

Explanation: A strong core is essential for stability and posture. This workout targets the core muscles, helping you build strength in the abdominal and lower back regions.

Tips: Perform core exercises with controlled movements and proper form. Incorporate these exercises into your routine 2-3 times a week for optimal results.

Flexibility Workout:

Explanation: Flexibility is key to maintaining joint health and mobility. This routine focuses on stretching exercises that improve flexibility and reduce the risk of injury.

Tips: Perform flexibility exercises after a warm-up or as part of your cool-down routine. Focus on slow, gentle stretches and avoid pushing your body beyond its comfort zone.

Resistance Band Workout:

Explanation: Resistance bands provide a gentle yet effective way to build muscle strength. This workout incorporates resistance band exercises to target various muscle groups.

Tips: Choose the appropriate resistance level for your fitness level. Gradually increase resistance as you progress. Maintain proper form and controlled movements during exercises.

Bosu/Exercise Ball Workout:

Explanation: The Bosu ball and exercise ball add an element of instability to exercises, engaging core and stabilizing muscles. This workout utilizes these tools for a balanced workout routine.

Tips: Start with basic exercises on the Bosu or exercise ball to build stability and confidence. Use proper safety precautions and consider professional guidance if you're new to these tools.

Arm Strength Workout:

Explanation: Upper body strength is crucial for everyday activities. This workout focuses on exercises that target the arms, shoulders, and chest, helping you build functional strength.

Tips: Start with light weights or resistance bands, gradually increasing the resistance as you progress. Pay attention to proper form to prevent strain or injury.

These workout routines offer a well-rounded fitness approach for seniors, promoting strength, balance, flexibility, and overall health. Choose the routines that align with your goals and abilities, and remember to consult with a healthcare provider or fitness professional if you have specific health concerns or limitations. Consistency and gradual progression are key to reaping the benefits of these routines.

The Best Exercises for Seniors

Exercise is a crucial component of a healthy lifestyle for seniors, but it's important to choose activities that are safe, effective, and tailored to individual needs. Here are some of the best exercises for seniors to consider:

1. Water Aerobics:

Explanation: Water aerobics have gained popularity among seniors due to their low-impact nature. Exercising in water is gentle on joints, making it ideal for those with arthritis or joint pain. The natural resistance of water eliminates the need for weights, making it great for strength training. Water aerobics improve strength, flexibility, and balance with minimal stress on the body.

Great exercises for seniors: Aqua jogging, flutter kicking, leg lifts, standing water push-ups, arm curls.

2. Chair Yoga:

Explanation: Chair yoga is a low-impact form of exercise that improves muscle strength, mobility, balance, and flexibility, all vital aspects of senior health. It is accessible and places less strain on muscles, joints, and bones compared to conventional yoga.

Great chair yoga exercises for seniors: Overhead stretch, seated cow stretch, seated cat stretch, seated mountain pose, seated twist.

3. Resistance Band Workouts:

Explanation: Resistance bands add gentle resistance to workouts, making them suitable for seniors. These bands are user-friendly and cost-effective, making them ideal for home exercise. Resistance band workouts strengthen the core, improving posture, mobility, and balance.

Great resistance band exercises for seniors: Leg press, triceps press, lateral raise, bicep curl, band pull apart.

4. Pilates:

Explanation: Pilates is a low-impact exercise that emphasizes breathing, alignment, concentration, and core strength. It often involves mats and accessories like pilates balls. Pilates enhances balance, core strength, and flexibility in older adults.

Great pilates exercises for seniors: Mermaid movement, side circles, food slides, step-ups, leg circle.

5. Walking:

Explanation: Walking is one of the least stressful and accessible forms of exercise. It promotes cardiovascular health, strengthens muscles, and lowers the risk of various health issues, including heart disease, stroke, diabetes, and colon cancer.

Ideas for walking exercises for seniors: Find a moderate trail through a park, participate in a walk-friendly race, walk the perimeter of a familiar building, listen to audiobooks or music during your walk.

6. Body Weight Workouts:
Explanation: Muscle loss can be a concern for seniors. Body weight workouts are effective in countering muscle atrophy. They are affordable and require minimal equipment, usually just workout clothes and a mat.

Great body weight workouts for seniors: Squats to chair, step-up, bird dog, lying hip bridges, side-lying circles.

7. Dumbbell Strength Training:

Explanation: Strength training is beneficial for seniors as it can alleviate symptoms of various health conditions and improve metabolism and glucose control. Dumbbells are suitable for isolating muscle groups while enhancing balance and flexibility.

Ideal dumbbell workouts for seniors: Bent-over row, tricep extension, bicep curl, overhead press, front raise.

Exercises Seniors Should Avoid:

It's important for seniors to avoid certain exercises that may strain their joints, muscles, or balance. High-intensity workouts designed for younger adults may not be suitable for seniors with specific health concerns. These exercises should be approached with caution:

High-impact activities like running or intense aerobics.

Heavy weightlifting without proper supervision and form.

Exercises that involve quick, jerking movements Extreme flexibility exercises that push joints beyond their limits.

Before starting any new exercise regimen, seniors should consult with a healthcare provider or fitness professional to ensure that the chosen exercises are safe and appropriate for their individual health status and fitness level. Safety should always be a top priority when engaging in physical activity as a senior.

CHAPTER SIX - COOLING-DOWN EXERCISES

After a workout, it's essential to allow your body to cool down properly. Cooling down helps in preventing post-workout discomfort and promotes a gradual return to your normal heart rate and breathing. Here are some effective cooling-down exercises and practices:

1. Pre-Cool Before the Workout:

Before you even begin your workout, consider pre-cooling. This practice helps slow the rate of your body temperature increase during exercise and can enhance your performance. Pre-cooling methods include hydrating with cold drinks at least two hours before your workout, spending time in an air-conditioned room, or having cooling packs on hand.

2. Stretch It Out Post-Workout:

After your workout, don't rush to the shower. Take at least ten minutes to walk and stretch. This cooldown period allows your heart rate to gradually decrease, preventing post-workout sweats and helping you avoid lightheadedness.

3. Take a Hot-and-Cold Shower:

Once you've completed your cooldown exercises, take a shower. However, don't make it cold the entire time. Research has shown that alternating between hot and cold water after exercise can lead to a significant reduction in heart rate and blood lactate levels. This can aid in your recovery process.

4. Apply Skin-Cooling Lotion:

After your shower, consider using a lotion that contains cooling properties like menthol. These lotions can provide a refreshing sensation to your skin, similar to how aloe vera soothes sunburn. Look for products designed to hydrate and cool your skin, leaving you feeling refreshed.

5. Enjoy Peppermint Tea—Hot or Cold:

Peppermint tea can help cool your body, although the mechanism is somewhat counterintuitive. In dry, hot climates, drinking hot tea can trigger a sweating response, helping you cool down. However, the cooling effect occurs when the sweat evaporates, so this method may not be as effective in humid climates. If you're in a humid environment, opt for iced tea with peppermint, which contains menthol—a cooling compound.

By incorporating these cooling-down exercises and practices into your post-workout routine, you can enhance your recovery and ensure a more comfortable return to your daily activities. Remember that proper cooling down is essential for overall workout safety and effectiveness.

- Staying Fit as You Age

Remaining physically active as you age is not only beneficial but essential for maintaining independence, preventing health issues, and ensuring a high quality of life. Here are some key considerations for staying fit as you grow older:

1. Regular Exercise: Aim to exercise at least three times a week. Regular physical activity improves your strength and balance, increases energy levels, enhances mood, and even boosts brain function. Activities such as biking, walking, dancing, tennis, yoga, and fitness classes can all contribute to a healthy lifestyle.

2. Independence: Regular exercise is a key factor in preserving independence in older adults. Those who exercise regularly are less likely to rely on others for daily tasks. If maintaining self-sufficiency is important to you, prioritize regular physical activity.

3. Flexibility: Stretching and yoga are excellent for maintaining your range of motion. This flexibility helps you perform daily tasks like reaching into cabinets, bending to pick up objects, and improving overall posture while reducing stiffness.

4. Balance: Falls are a significant concern among seniors, with many resulting in serious injuries. Regular exercise can reduce the risk of falls by 25%. Activities like yoga, Tai Chi, one-foot balance exercises, and tandem walking can challenge and improve your walking abilities, in addition to promoting healthy feet.

5. Strength Training: As you age, you naturally lose about 10% of your general strength every decade. Strength training, whether with resistance bands, light weights, or body weight exercises like pushups and planks, can help mitigate muscle mass loss and increase overall strength.

6. Endurance: Endurance is the ability to exert yourself and remain active for longer periods while recovering from fatigue, injury, or illness. Improved endurance allows you to perform daily tasks more efficiently. Activities like swimming, water aerobics, and walking (aiming for 10,000 steps a day) can help enhance your endurance.

7. Silver Sneakers: Many health insurance programs, including Medicare, offer a "Silver Sneakers" plan for seniors aged 65 and older. This program provides free health and fitness classes, both online and in-person, tailored to older adults. Be sure to check your insurance benefits to see if you are eligible for this valuable resource.

Incorporating these principles into your daily life can help you enjoy a healthier, more active, and more independent lifestyle as you age. Regular physical activity is an investment in your long-term well-being and vitality.

Muscle Recovery in Seniors

Muscle recovery in seniors is a crucial aspect of maintaining physical health and well-being as one ages. Understanding how seniors recover and the various ways in which muscles recover can help ensure that older individuals can continue to engage in regular physical activities and lead a fulfilling life. Here's a professional explanation:

Muscle Recovery in Seniors

As people age, their bodies undergo natural changes, including a decline in muscle mass and strength. Muscle recovery in seniors is the process by which their muscles repair and adapt after physical activity or exercise. This recovery is essential for several reasons:

Recovery from Exercise: After engaging in physical activity, especially resistance or strength training, muscles experience micro-tears. Muscle recovery allows these tears to heal, resulting in stronger and more resilient muscles.

Reducing Soreness: Muscle recovery helps reduce post-exercise soreness and stiffness, which can be more pronounced in seniors due to age-related changes in muscle tissue.

Maintaining Functionality: Effective muscle recovery supports seniors in maintaining their ability to perform daily activities, from walking and climbing stairs to lifting objects and maintaining balance.

Ways in Which Our Muscles Recover

Rest and Sleep: Adequate rest and sleep are fundamental to muscle recovery. During deep sleep stages, the body releases growth hormone, which plays a key role in repairing and rebuilding muscles. Seniors should prioritize getting 7-9 hours of quality sleep each night.

Nutrition: Proper nutrition is vital for muscle recovery. Seniors should ensure they consume an adequate amount of protein, which provides essential amino acids necessary for muscle repair. A balanced diet rich in vitamins and minerals also supports overall health and recovery.

Hydration: Staying hydrated is critical for muscle function and recovery. Dehydration can lead to muscle cramps and impair the body's ability to repair muscle tissue. Seniors should drink plenty of water throughout the day.

Stretching and Flexibility: Incorporating stretching exercises into a fitness routine can enhance muscle recovery by improving flexibility and reducing muscle tightness. Activities like yoga and static stretching can be particularly beneficial for seniors.

Active Recovery: Engaging in light, low-impact physical activities on rest days can promote blood flow to the muscles, aiding in recovery. Activities like walking or swimming can help prevent stiffness and promote healing.

Massage and Foam Rolling: Massage therapy and self-myofascial release techniques using foam rollers can help alleviate muscle tension and improve circulation, supporting muscle recovery.

Professional Guidance: Seniors can benefit from consulting with healthcare professionals or physical therapists who specialize in geriatric care. These experts can provide personalized advice on exercise routines and recovery strategies tailored to individual needs.

In conclusion, muscle recovery is a vital component of maintaining physical function and overall well-being in seniors. By prioritizing rest, nutrition, hydration, and appropriate exercise, older individuals can optimize muscle recovery and continue to lead active and independent lives as they age.

Conclusion

In conclusion, this comprehensive guide explores the world of strength training and exercise for seniors, emphasizing the importance of staying active and fit as we age. We've covered various aspects, from the benefits of strength training and different approaches to exercises to the importance of developing a workout habit and effective cooling-down techniques. Additionally, we've highlighted the best exercises for seniors and how muscle recovery plays a crucial role in maintaining physical health.

For seniors, staying active isn't just a choice; it's a key factor in maintaining independence, preventing health problems, and enhancing overall well-being. Regular exercise, tailored to individual needs and capabilities, can improve strength, flexibility, balance, and endurance. It's a powerful tool for aging gracefully and enjoying a high quality of life.

Furthermore, we've discussed some precautions, such as exercises to avoid, and encouraged seniors to consult with healthcare professionals or specialists for personalized guidance.

Remember that age should never be a barrier to pursuing a healthy, active lifestyle. With the right knowledge, dedication, and support, seniors can continue to lead fulfilling lives, staying fit and strong as they age. It's never too late to start, and the benefits of regular exercise are well worth the effort. So, take the first step on your fitness journey and embrace the path to a healthier, happier, and more vibrant senior life.

FITNESS PROGRESS JOURNAL

Date: ____/____/____   ____/____/____

Body Parts	Before	After

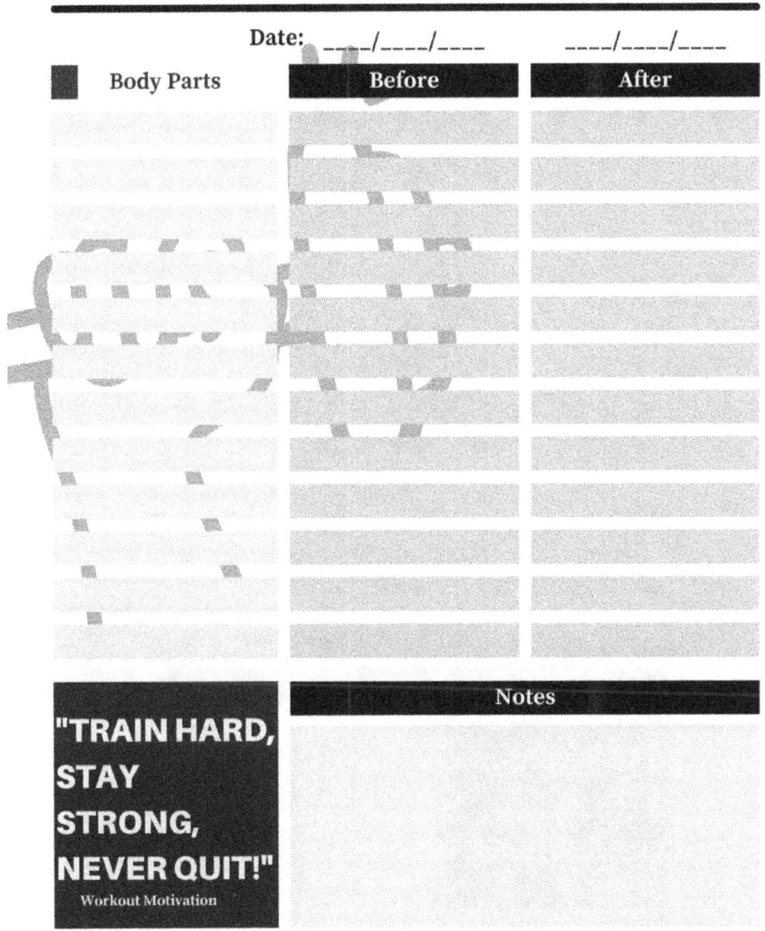

"TRAIN HARD, STAY STRONG, NEVER QUIT!"
Workout Motivation

Notes

FITNESS PROGRESS JOURNAL

Date: ____/____/____   ____/____/____

Body Parts	Before	After

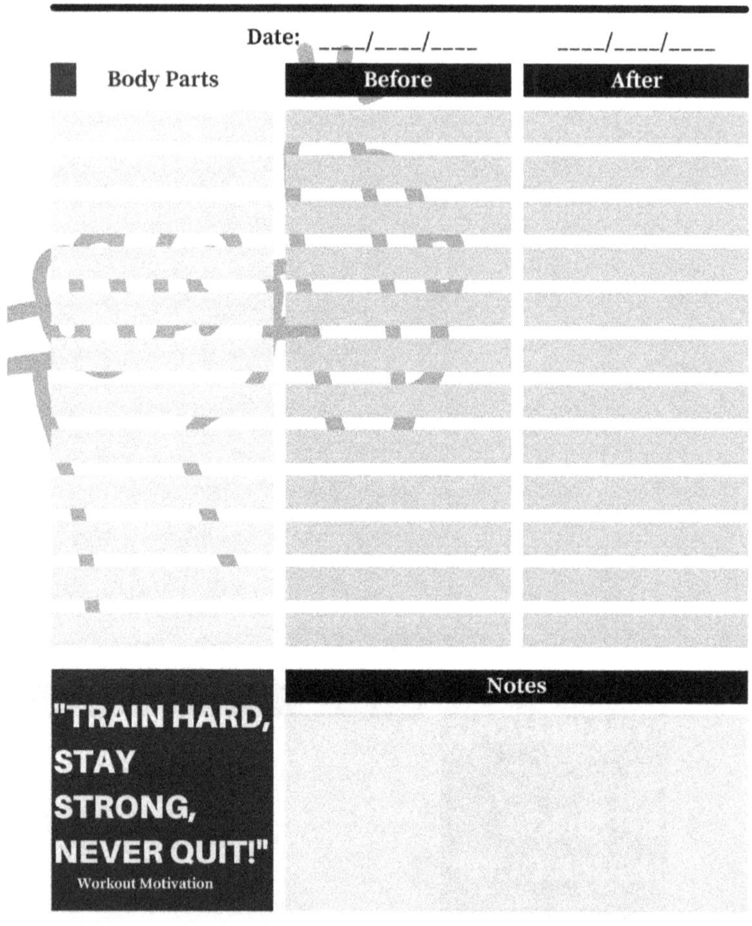

	Notes
"TRAIN HARD, STAY STRONG, NEVER QUIT!" Workout Motivation	

FITNESS PROGRESS JOURNAL

Date: ____/____/____   ____/____/____

Body Parts	Before	After

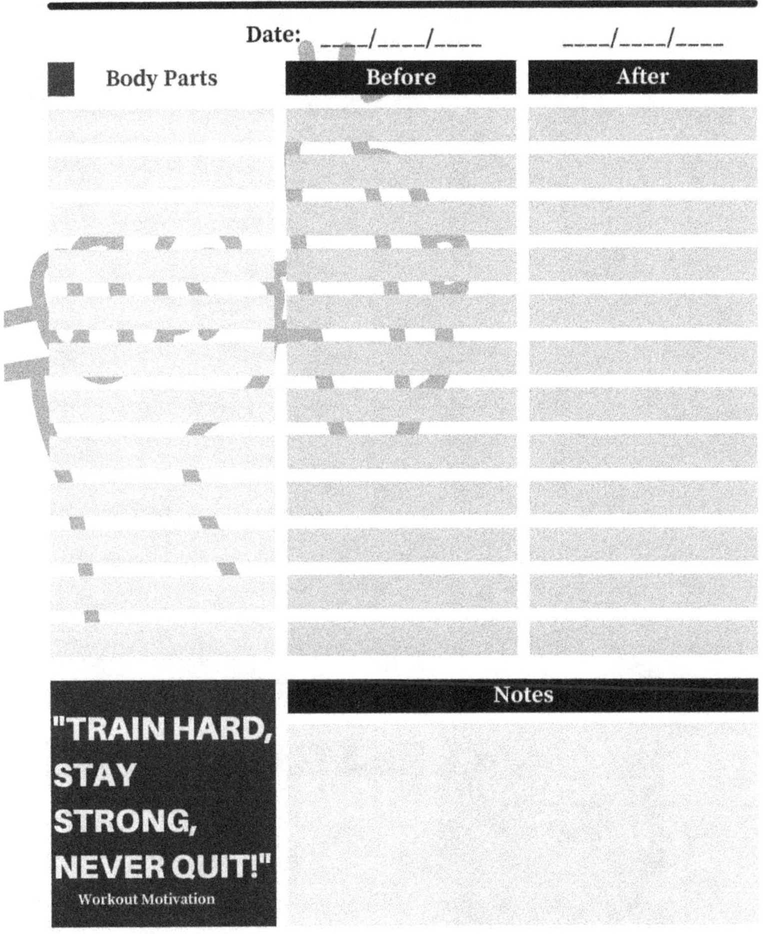

"TRAIN HARD, STAY STRONG, NEVER QUIT!"
Workout Motivation

Notes

FITNESS PROGRESS JOURNAL

Date: ____/____/____   ____/____/____

Body Parts	Before	After

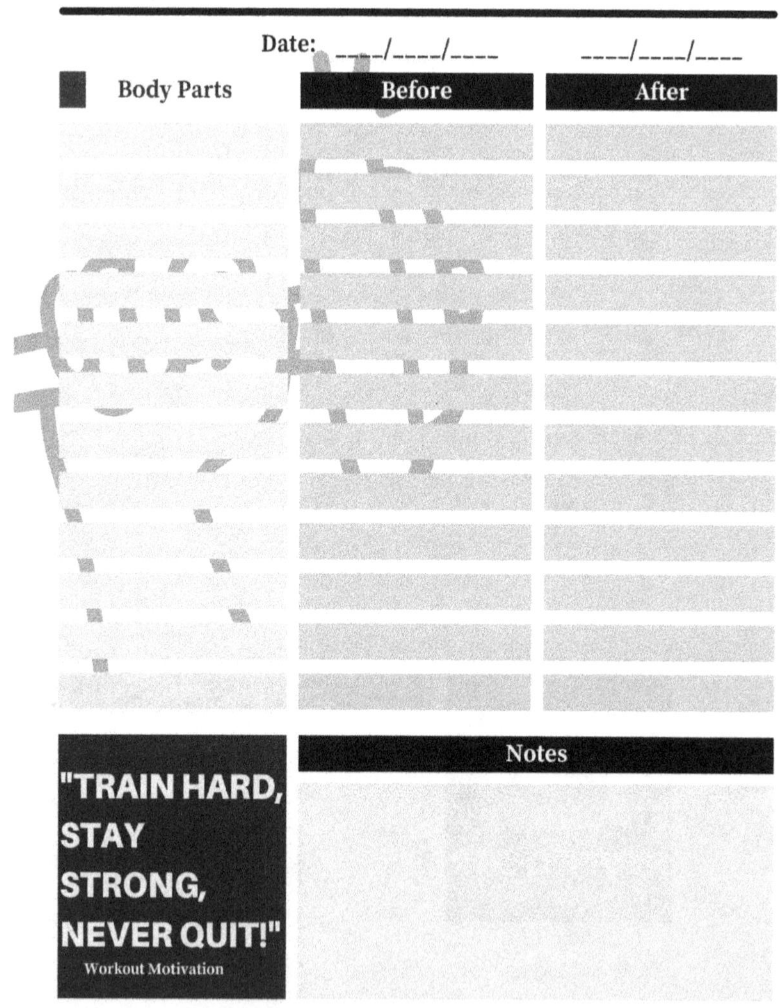

"TRAIN HARD, STAY STRONG, NEVER QUIT!"
Workout Motivation

Notes

FITNESS PROGRESS JOURNAL

Date: ____/____/____   ____/____/____

Body Parts	Before	After

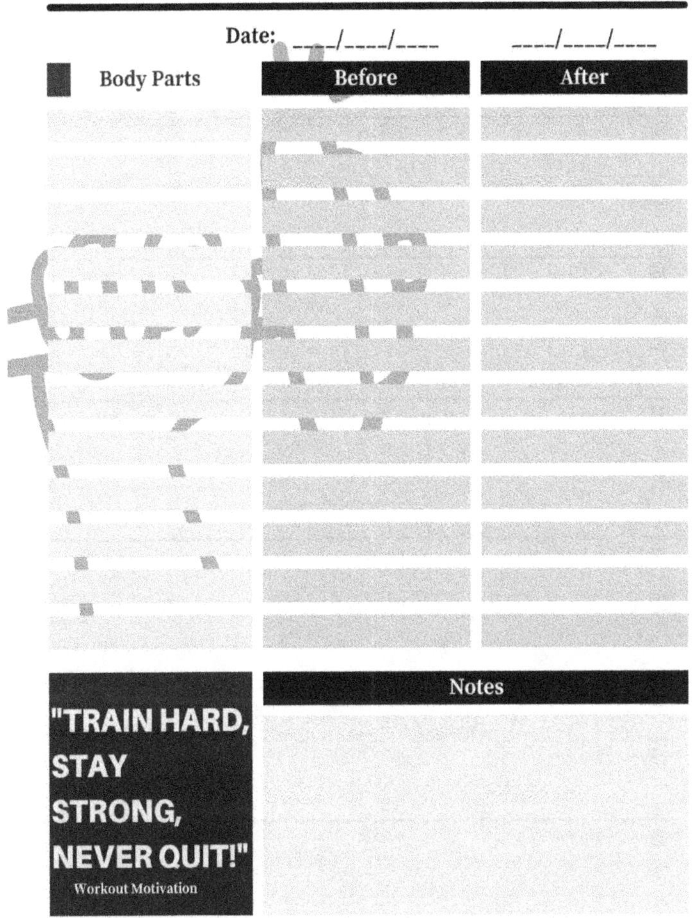

"TRAIN HARD, STAY STRONG, NEVER QUIT!"	Notes
Workout Motivation	

MY WEEKLY WORKOUT LOG

MON

	Activities	Tracker		Notes
		Sets :	Date:	
		Reps :	Weight:	
		Calories :	Distance:	

TUE

	Activities	Tracker		Notes
		Sets :	Date:	
		Reps :	Weight:	
		Calories :	Distance:	

WED

	Activities	Tracker		Notes
		Sets :	Date:	
		Reps :	Weight:	
		Calories :	Distance:	

THU

	Activities	Tracker		Notes
		Sets :	Date:	
		Reps :	Weight:	
		Calories :	Distance:	

FRI

	Activities	Tracker		Notes
		Sets :	Date:	
		Reps :	Weight:	
		Calories :	Distance:	

SAT

	Activities	Tracker		Notes
		Sets :	Date:	
		Reps :	Weight:	
		Calories :	Distance:	

SUN

	Activities	Tracker		Notes
		Sets :	Date:	
		Reps :	Weight:	
		Calories :	Distance:	

MY WEEKLY WORKOUT LOG

MON

Activities

Tracker
Sets :
Date:
Reps :
Weight:
Calories :
Distance:

Notes

TUE

Activities

Tracker
Sets :
Date:
Reps :
Weight:
Calories :
Distance:

Notes

WED

Activities

Tracker
Sets :
Date:
Reps :
Weight:
Calories :
Distance:

Notes

THU

Activities

Tracker
Sets :
Date:
Reps :
Weight:
Calories :
Distance:

Notes

FRI

Activities

Tracker
Sets :
Date:
Reps :
Weight:
Calories :
Distance:

Notes

SAT

Activities

Tracker
Sets :
Date:
Reps :
Weight:
Calories :
Distance:

Notes

SUN

Activities

Tracker
Sets :
Date:
Reps :
Weight:
Calories :
Distance:

Notes

MY WEEKLY WORKOUT LOG

MON
Activities	Tracker		Notes
	Sets :	Date:	
	Reps :	Weight:	
	Calories :	Distance:	

TUE
Activities	Tracker		Notes
	Sets :	Date:	
	Reps :	Weight:	
	Calories :	Distance:	

WED
Activities	Tracker		Notes
	Sets :	Date:	
	Reps :	Weight:	
	Calories :	Distance:	

THU
Activities	Tracker		Notes
	Sets :	Date:	
	Reps :	Weight:	
	Calories :	Distance:	

FRI
Activities	Tracker		Notes
	Sets :	Date:	
	Reps :	Weight:	
	Calories :	Distance:	

SAT
Activities	Tracker		Notes
	Sets :	Date:	
	Reps :	Weight:	
	Calories :	Distance:	

SUN
Activities	Tracker		Notes
	Sets :	Date:	
	Reps :	Weight:	
	Calories :	Distance:	

MY WEEKLY WORKOUT LOG

	Activities	Tracker		Notes
MON		Sets :	Date:	
		Reps :	Weight:	
		Calories :	Distance:	

	Activities	Tracker		Notes
TUE		Sets :	Date:	
		Reps :	Weight:	
		Calories :	Distance:	

	Activities	Tracker		Notes
WED		Sets :	Date:	
		Reps :	Weight:	
		Calories :	Distance:	

	Activities	Tracker		Notes
THU		Sets :	Date:	
		Reps :	Weight:	
		Calories :	Distance:	

	Activities	Tracker		Notes
FRI		Sets :	Date:	
		Reps :	Weight:	
		Calories :	Distance:	

	Activities	Tracker		Notes
SAT		Sets :	Date:	
		Reps :	Weight:	
		Calories :	Distance:	

	Activities	Tracker		Notes
SUN		Sets :	Date:	
		Reps :	Weight:	
		Calories :	Distance:	

MY WEEKLY WORKOUT LOG

MON

Activities	Tracker		Notes
	Sets :	Date:	
	Reps :	Weight:	
	Calories :	Distance:	

TUE

Activities	Tracker		Notes
	Sets :	Date:	
	Reps :	Weight:	
	Calories :	Distance:	

WED

Activities	Tracker		Notes
	Sets :	Date:	
	Reps :	Weight:	
	Calories :	Distance:	

THU

Activities	Tracker		Notes
	Sets :	Date:	
	Reps :	Weight:	
	Calories :	Distance:	

FRI

Activities	Tracker		Notes
	Sets :	Date:	
	Reps :	Weight:	
	Calories :	Distance:	

SAT

Activities	Tracker		Notes
	Sets :	Date:	
	Reps :	Weight:	
	Calories :	Distance:	

SUN

Activities	Tracker		Notes
	Sets :	Date:	
	Reps :	Weight:	
	Calories :	Distance:	

FOOD TRACKER

Date	Breakfast	Lunch	Dinner	Snack
SUN				
MON				
TUE				
WED				
THU				
FRI				
SAT				

Notes	Target Weight

FOOD TRACKER

Date	Breakfast	Lunch	Dinner	Snack
SUN				
MON				
TUE				
WED				
THU				
FRI				
SAT				

Notes	Target Weight

FOOD TRACKER

Date	Breakfast	Lunch	Dinner	Snack
SUN				
MON				
TUE				
WED				
THU				
FRI				
SAT				

Notes

Target Weight

FOOD TRACKER

Date	Breakfast	Lunch	Dinner	Snack
SUN				
MON				
TUE				
WED				
THU				
FRI				
SAT				

Notes	Target Weight

FOOD TRACKER

Date	Breakfast	Lunch	Dinner	Snack
SUN				
MON				
TUE				
WED				
THU				
FRI				
SAT				

Notes	Target Weight

FOOD TRACKER

Date	Breakfast	Lunch	Dinner	Snack
SUN				
MON				
TUE				
WED				
THU				
FRI				
SAT				

Notes	Target Weight

WEIGHT TRACKER

MARCH

Week 1	Week 2	Week 3	Week 4
.lbs	.lbs	.lbs	.lbs

APRIL

Week 1	Week 2	Week 3	Week 4
.lbs	.lbs	.lbs	.lbs

MAY

Week 1	Week 2	Week 3	Week 4
.lbs	.lbs	.lbs	.lbs

Notes	Before	After
	.lbs	.lbs

TARGET WEIGHT

.lbs

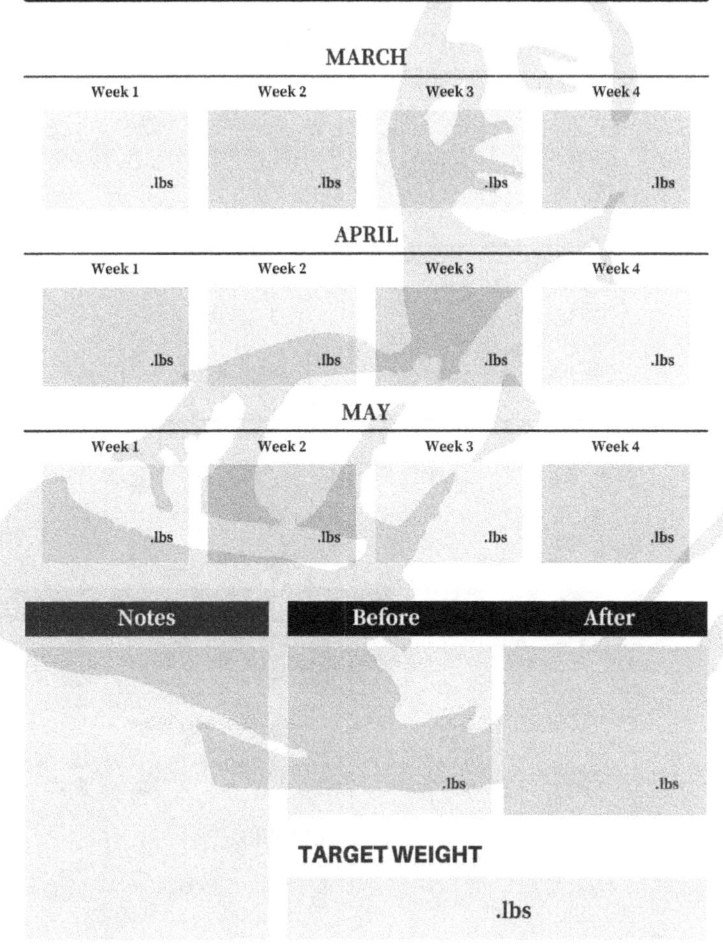

WEIGHT TRACKER

MARCH

Week 1	Week 2	Week 3	Week 4
.lbs	.lbs	.lbs	.lbs

APRIL

Week 1	Week 2	Week 3	Week 4
.lbs	.lbs	.lbs	.lbs

MAY

Week 1	Week 2	Week 3	Week 4
.lbs	.lbs	.lbs	.lbs

Notes	Before	After
	.lbs	.lbs

TARGET WEIGHT

.lbs

WEIGHT TRACKER

MARCH

Week 1	Week 2	Week 3	Week 4
.lbs	.lbs	.lbs	.lbs

APRIL

Week 1	Week 2	Week 3	Week 4
.lbs	.lbs	.lbs	.lbs

MAY

Week 1	Week 2	Week 3	Week 4
.lbs	.lbs	.lbs	.lbs

Notes	Before	After
	.lbs	.lbs

TARGET WEIGHT

.lbs

WEIGHT TRACKER

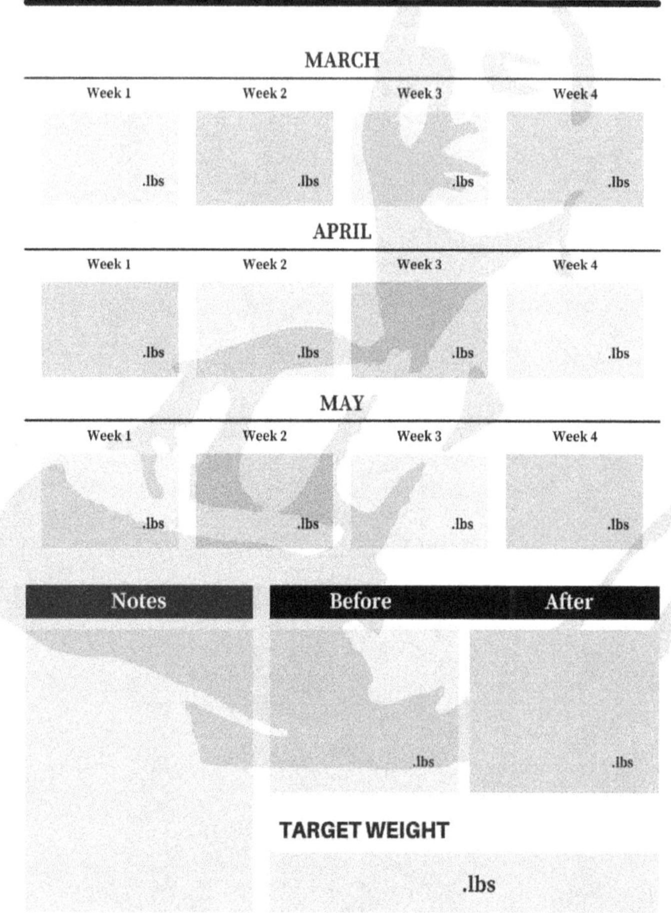

MARCH

Week 1	Week 2	Week 3	Week 4
.lbs	.lbs	.lbs	.lbs

APRIL

Week 1	Week 2	Week 3	Week 4
.lbs	.lbs	.lbs	.lbs

MAY

Week 1	Week 2	Week 3	Week 4
.lbs	.lbs	.lbs	.lbs

Notes	Before	After
	.lbs	.lbs

TARGET WEIGHT

.lbs

WEIGHT TRACKER

MARCH

Week 1	Week 2	Week 3	Week 4
.lbs	.lbs	.lbs	.lbs

APRIL

Week 1	Week 2	Week 3	Week 4
.lbs	.lbs	.lbs	.lbs

MAY

Week 1	Week 2	Week 3	Week 4
.lbs	.lbs	.lbs	.lbs

Notes	Before	After
	.lbs	.lbs

TARGET WEIGHT

.lbs

WEIGHT TRACKER

MARCH

Week 1	Week 2	Week 3	Week 4
.lbs	.lbs	.lbs	.lbs

APRIL

Week 1	Week 2	Week 3	Week 4
.lbs	.lbs	.lbs	.lbs

MAY

Week 1	Week 2	Week 3	Week 4
.lbs	.lbs	.lbs	.lbs

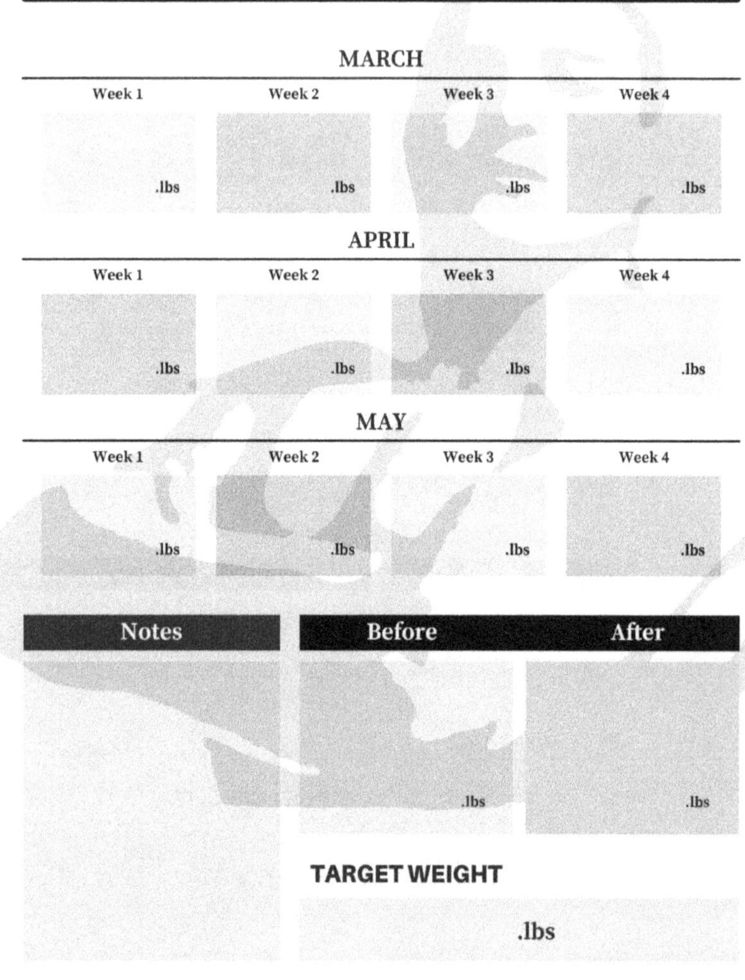

Notes	Before	After
	.lbs	.lbs

TARGET WEIGHT

.lbs